Alzheimer's Diet
Cookbook for seniors

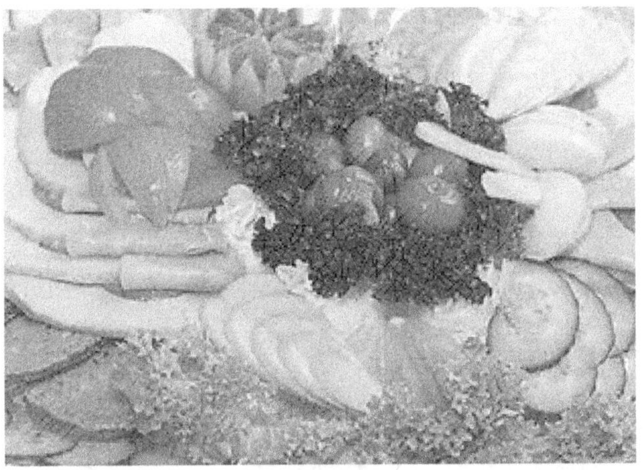

A 30-Day Alzheimer's solution and Lifestyle Guide to Prevent Cognitive Decline, Memory disorder and Stimulate the Mind

Mattie Morgan

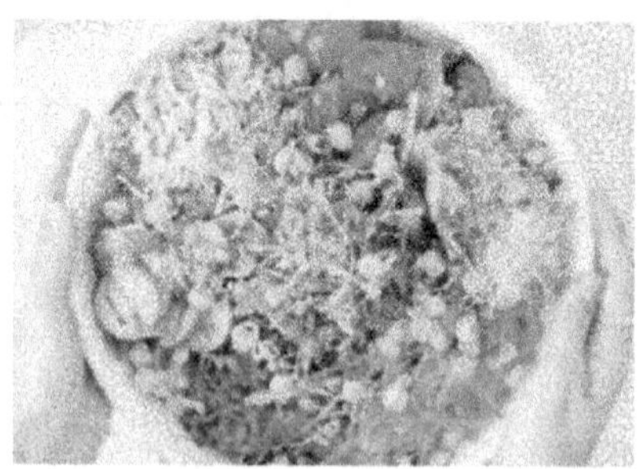

Table of Contents

Introduction

Sharon had always treasured her memories—until they began to slip through her fingers like sand. Alzheimer's had crept into her life, taking parts of her past and leaving her befuddled. Her once-vivacious attitude had withered as she teetered on the brink of dementia.

Hope glowed softly in a simple diet plan she discovered in a forgotten corner of the internet (my article). She accepted the program with unyielding dedication, determined to reject the horrible doom that loomed above her. Her regular companions were organic greens, omega-rich almonds, and antioxidant-rich fruits. She said goodbye to refined sweets and accepted herbal teas as her elixir.

Days became weeks, and a subtle alteration swept across her being. Her thoughts began to awaken gradually, like a fading flower rejuvenated by soft rain. Laughter with friends, the aroma of her grandmother's food, and the warmth of her children's hug returned from the fog.

Each new day blossomed like a flowering triumphant story. Sharon, despite all odds, made her way out of the maze of oblivion. Her eyes twinkled with recognition, and her formerly hesitant grin now emanated a calm strength—a testament to her tenacity and the power of nourishing both body and soul. The woman who had almost succumbed to dementia reemerged, her spirit unbreakable, her memories a treasure once more.

Alzheimer's disease is a progressive neurological ailment that robs people of their memories, cognitive ability, and, finally, independence. This disorder, first recognized by Dr. Alois Alzheimer in 1906, generally affects elderly persons; however, early-onset cases do arise.

Alzheimer's disease is distinguished by the formation of aberrant protein deposits—beta-amyloid plaques and tau tangles—which lead to the slow degeneration of brain cells. This deterioration impairs neuronal connection, weakening cognitive skills such as memory, thinking, and behavior.

Its gradual beginning is generally accompanied by modest memory loss, disorientation, and trouble executing familiar activities.

As the condition progresses, people may struggle with language, have mood changes, and have difficulty recognizing loved ones. Alzheimer's disease has a significant impact not just on the affected person but also on their caregivers and family, needing significant emotional, physical, and financial assistance.

Alzheimer's disease currently has no cure. However, current research efforts are aimed at unraveling its intricacies, identifying new therapies, and devising interventions to alleviate symptoms and slow the course of the disease.

Early detection, diets, lifestyle changes, and some drugs may provide temporary relief, emphasizing the significance of raising awareness, providing support, and continuing research in the battle against this tough neurological disorder.

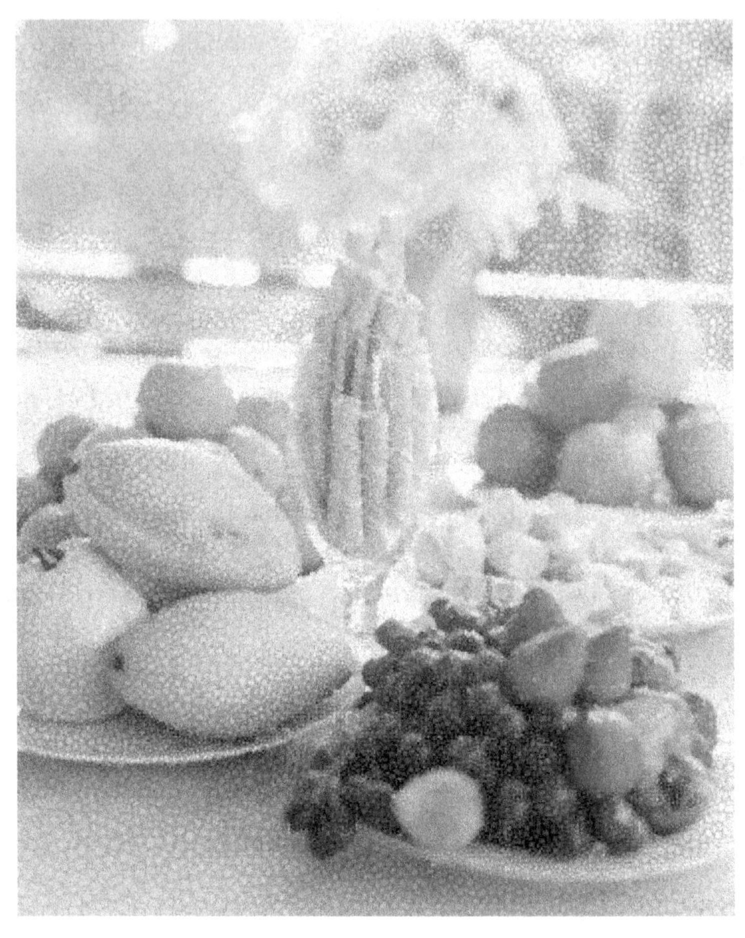

Chapter 1: Overview of Alzheimer's and Its Impact on seniors

Alzheimer's disease, a kind of dementia, has as major impact on the elderly, gradually degrading their cognitive capacities and changing their everyday lives. Alzheimer's disease is the most prevalent form of dementia, affecting memory, thinking, and behavior and offering enormous problems to both patients and their loved ones.

The illness progresses in phases, with mild symptoms such as forgetfulness and trouble doing routine tasks at first. It progresses to moderate and severe phases over time, significantly limiting a person's ability to speak, identify their environment, and do even simple activities.

The impact on elders is complex. It has an impact on their independence, requiring more assistance with daily functions such as washing, dressing, and eating. Individuals may struggle to recall essential information, faces, or even their history as memory loss worsens, producing frustration, worry, and loneliness.

The emotional toll on seniors is significant, frequently resulting in bewilderment, mood swings, and personality changes. It also places a strain on families and caregivers, requiring 24-hour care, compassion, and understanding.

The financial burden is also enormous, with Alzheimer's requiring extensive healthcare bills and long-term care and sometimes forcing people to retire sooner than intended, jeopardizing their financial stability.

Alzheimer's disease has a severe impact on the lives of seniors, threatening their independence, straining relationships, and requiring comprehensive support systems to traverse the complicated and demanding journey it presents.

Anyone presenting symptoms resembling dementia should promptly consult a healthcare professional. **What are the indications of Alzheimer's disease?** The symptoms of Alzheimer's (AD) differ depending on the disease stage.

Generally, AD symptoms encompass a gradual decline in one or more of the following:

- Memory

- Reasoning and managing complex tasks

- Language

- Comprehending spatial relationships

- Behavior and personality

Individuals experiencing memory loss or other Alzheimer's symptoms may struggle to acknowledge their cognitive decline. These signs might be more apparent to their loved ones. It's crucial for anyone exhibiting dementia-like symptoms to seek medical attention promptly.

Mild Stage Symptoms of Alzheimer's: The early stage reveals memory lapses, particularly forgetting recent events, locations, or names. Other signs include:

- Difficulty in articulating thoughts

- Increased misplacement of objects

- Challenges in planning or organization

- Struggles in problem-solving

- Slower completion of routine tasks

Those in the mild stage typically recognize familiar faces and navigate known places without much trouble.

Moderate Stage Symptoms of Alzheimer's: This phase, often prolonged, necessitates increased care. Symptoms include:

- Heightened memory loss and confusion, forgetting personal details or recent events

- Growing disorientation about time, seasons, and location

- Worsening short-term memory

- Difficulty recognizing family and friends

- Repeatedly sharing thoughts or events

- Struggles with basic arithmetic

- Needing assistance with personal care

- Heightened personality changes, agitation, depression, or anxiety

- Development of unfounded suspicions (delusions)

- Onset of urinary or bowel incontinence

- Sleep disturbances and wandering

Severe Stage Symptoms of Alzheimer's: In the final stage, symptoms are severe, requiring extensive care. At this stage, individuals may:

- Experience almost complete memory loss

- Show unawareness of surroundings

- Depend on assistance for daily activities like eating, sitting, and walking

- Lose communication ability to a few words or phrases

- Become vulnerable to infections, particularly pneumonia and skin infections, necessitating hospice care for comfort.

Is Alzheimer's Hereditary? Researchers haven't pinpointed why some people develop Alzheimer's while others don't. However, they've identified risk factors, including genetics. Carrying the APOE ε4 form of the apolipoprotein E gene increases the risk but doesn't guarantee the condition. Having a first-degree relative with Alzheimer's raises the risk by 10% to 30%. Individuals with multiple siblings having late-onset Alzheimer's have higher risks.

Prevention: Certain risk factors like age and genetics are uncontrollable, but managing others might reduce risk. Strategies include:

- Mental stimulation: Engage in brain-stimulating activities.

- Physical activity: Exercise enhances brain cell health.

- Social engagement: Interact regularly with peers.

- Healthy diet: Consume antioxidants and moderate alcohol.

- Preventive measures: Manage factors like high blood pressure, cholesterol, diabetes, obesity, depression, and avoid smoking.

The Role of Diet in Alzheimer's Management

Diet has a significant impact on Alzheimer's disease progression, treatment, and even potential reversal. While there is no cure, evidence shows that certain dietary patterns may help to alleviate symptoms, decrease the progression of the illness, and lower the chance of developing Alzheimer's.

Brain-Healthy Nutrients: Certain nutrients found in fruits, vegetables, nuts, and fatty fish, such as omega-3 fatty acids, antioxidants (such as vitamin E and C), and flavonoids, are thought to boost brain function.

These elements have the potential to counteract inflammation and oxidative stress, which may aid with cognitive maintenance.

The Mediterranean diet, which is high in fruits, vegetables, whole grains, fish, olive oil, and moderate wine consumption, has been demonstrated to reduce the risk of cognitive impairment. It emphasizes healthy fats, antioxidants, and phytochemicals, which may help prevent Alzheimer's disease.

Low-Sugar and Processed Meals: Sugar and processed meals have been linked to inflammation, which may lead to cognitive impairment. Reducing these items in the diet may help manage Alzheimer's symptoms.

Weight Control and Heart Health: Obesity, diabetes, and high blood pressure are all linked to an increased risk of Alzheimer's. A diet focused on maintaining a healthy weight and supporting heart health may indirectly help reduce Alzheimer's risk.

Intermittent fasting and a ketogenic diet (low-carb, high-fat): A new study reveals that intermittent fasting and a ketogenic diet (low-carb, high-fat) may have neuroprotective advantages. They may improve brain function and perhaps help some people manage symptoms.

Chapter 2: Principles of a Brain-Boosting Diet

A brain-boosting diet focuses on providing vitamins and compounds to the brain that increase cognitive performance, guard against age-related decline, and promote general brain health. The following are the essential principles:

Nutrient-Rich Foods: Prioritize complete, nutrient-dense foods that supply critical vitamins, minerals, and antioxidants. Include colorful fruits and vegetables, whole grains, lean meats, healthy fats (such as those found in avocados, almonds, and olive oil), and omega-3 fatty acid sources such as fatty fish.

Omega-3 Fatty Acids: Include omega-3-rich foods like salmon, mackerel, walnuts, and flaxseeds in your diet. Omega-3 fatty acids are essential for brain health, boosting memory and cognitive function while perhaps lowering the risk of cognitive decline. Omega-3 fatty acids, notably EPA and DHA (docosahexaenoic acid), are essential for brain function.

They aid in maintaining neurotransmission, contribute to the construction of brain cell membranes, and may help decrease inflammation in the brain.

Antioxidant-Rich Foods: Consume antioxidant-rich foods such as berries, leafy greens, nuts, seeds, and colorful vegetables. Antioxidants protect the brain from oxidative stress and inflammation, hence improving general cognitive health.

B vitamins: B vitamins such as folate (B9), B6, and B12 are essential for cognitive function. They play a role in neurotransmitter synthesis and the control of homocysteine levels in the blood. Good sources include leafy greens, legumes, fortified cereals, and animal products such as eggs and dairy.

Phytochemicals: Plant compounds found in fruits, vegetables, nuts, and seeds, such as polyphenols and flavonoids, have antioxidant and anti-inflammatory activities. They may benefit brain health by shielding neurons from injury and lowering the risk of neurodegenerative disorders.

Healthy Fats: Make monounsaturated and polyunsaturated fats found in olive oil, avocados, nuts, and seeds a priority. These fats promote brain function by assisting in nerve signal transmission and maintaining healthy cell membranes.

Moderate Protein Intake: Consume lean protein sources such as poultry, fish, lentils, and tofu in moderation. Protein contains amino acids that are required for neurotransmitter formation, which aids cognitive function and mood modulation.

Glycemic Index Low carbs: To help balance blood sugar levels, choose complex carbs with a low glycemic index. Whole grains, legumes, and non-starchy veggies give a consistent source of energy to the brain while avoiding blood sugar spikes. High blood sugar levels have been linked to inflammation and a higher risk of cognitive impairment.

Hydration is important since dehydration can impair cognitive function. Drink enough water throughout the day to promote brain function and keep cognitive functioning at its peak.

Mindful Eating: Develop mindful eating habits that emphasize enjoying and appreciating each meal. Mindful eating can increase meal pleasure and help manage appetite and overall dietary intake.

Following these principles is critical since a brain-boosting diet attempts to offer the nutrients and chemicals needed to sustain brain function, defend against cognitive decline, and minimize the risk of neurodegenerative disorders.

The Science behind Brain-Healthy Foods

Brain-healthy foods are scientifically shown to protect brain cells from injury, support neurotransmitter function, reduce inflammation, and boost general brain health. Incorporating a mix of these items into a balanced diet may help to preserve cognitive function while also potentially lowering the risk of cognitive decline and neurodegenerative disorders such as Alzheimer's.

Here's a rundown of some essential points:

Magnesium: Magnesium, found in leafy greens, nuts, seeds, and whole grains, promotes cognitive function by promoting synaptic plasticity, which is essential for learning and memory. It is also involved in neurotransmission and the protection of neurons against excitotoxicity.

Zinc: found in oysters, red meat, chicken, and legumes, this mineral aids cognitive function, memory development, and learning. Zinc is involved in the regulation of neuronal transmission and may help guard against neurodegeneration.

Choline: Choline is a precursor of acetylcholine, a neurotransmitter important in memory and muscular function that may be found in eggs, liver, and some cereals. Adequate choline consumption promotes brain health, particularly throughout prenatal development and early infancy.

These nutrients help in the maintenance of brain cell structure and function, neurotransmitter generation, protection against oxidative stress and inflammation, and general cognitive function and memory.

A well-balanced diet rich in nutrient-dense foods guarantees an appropriate intake of these critical nutrients for optimal brain function.

Choosing the Right Ingredients for Cognitive Support

Because specific nutrients and foods have been linked to brain health and cognitive function, choosing the proper elements for cognitive support is critical. A well-balanced diet high in essential nutrients may improve cognitive capacities, guard against age-related decline, and lower the risk of illnesses such as Alzheimer's disease.

Here's a guide to selecting the best ingredients for cognitive support:

Whole Foods Market: Place an emphasis on whole, less processed meals. Choose fresh fruits and vegetables, whole grains, lean meats, and healthy fats over processed foods.

Omega-3 Fatty Acids: For high omega-3 content, choose fatty fish such as salmon, trout, and mackerel. Flaxseeds, chia seeds, and walnuts are examples of plant-based sources.

Antioxidants: Choose colorful fruits and vegetables such as berries, leafy greens, tomatoes, and bell peppers. Antioxidants can also be found in dark chocolate, almonds, and green tea.

Curcumin: Add turmeric to meals or take curcumin supplements. It has anti-inflammatory and antioxidant effects.

Vitamin E: Increase your intake of vitamin E by eating foods like almonds, sunflower seeds, spinach, and avocados.

Vitamin D: Get as much sunlight as you can and eat vitamin D-rich foods such as fatty fish, fortified dairy products, and egg yolks.

B Vitamins: To maintain appropriate B vitamin consumption, consume a range of foods such as whole grains, legumes, leafy greens, eggs, and lean meats.

Cook with olive oil, nibble on nuts and seeds, and add avocados to salads or smoothies for healthy fats.

Colored variety: aim for a varied assortment of colored fruits and vegetables. Different hues frequently represent various important minerals and antioxidants.

Mindful Cooking Methods: Use cooking methods that preserve nutrients, such as steaming, baking, or softly sautéing meals. Excessive frying or overcooking should be avoided.

Reduce your intake of added sugars and processed foods: Reduce your use of sugary snacks, processed meals, and high-sugar beverages, which can have a detrimental impact on your cognitive health.

Moderation and Balance: Eat a well-balanced diet rich in nutrients. Balance different dietary categories and portion levels; moderation is essential.

Stay Hydrated: Drink lots of water since dehydration can impair cognitive function.

Chapter 3: Meal Planning Tips for seniors and Caregivers

Meal planning for seniors, especially when caregivers are involved, necessitates consideration of nutritional needs, dietary preferences, and, in certain cases, specific health issues. Here are some food preparation suggestions for seniors and caregivers:

Understand Your Dietary Needs: Seek advice from a dietician or healthcare expert if possible to assess the senior's nutritional needs in light of their health problems, medicines, and any dietary restrictions.

Balanced Nutrition: Make sure that your meals include a range of dietary categories, such as fruits and vegetables, lean proteins, whole grains, and healthy fats. This provides the necessary nutrients for good health.

Meal Preparation in Practice: Plan ahead of time. Set aside some time each week to organize your meals.

Make a meal plan or a weekly menu to help you with grocery shopping and meal preparation.

Simple and nutritious: Make the effort to make meals that are both simple and healthy. To save time and effort, use slow cookers, instant pots, or make meals in batches.

Aim for Variation: Include a variety of foods to keep meals interesting and provide a wide spectrum of nutrients.

Shopping for Groceries: Create a precise grocery list based on the meal plan to eliminate needless purchases and ensure that you have all the required products.

Shop wisely: choose fresh fruits and vegetables, whole grains, lean meats, and healthy fats. When fresh fruits and vegetables are unavailable, consider frozen or canned alternatives.

Consider Special Dietary Requirements: When preparing meals, keep any food allergies or intolerances in mind.

Health issues: Tailor meals to meet the requirements of seniors who have specific health issues, such as diabetes or high blood pressure. If required, choose low-sodium alternatives or meals with a regulated carbohydrate level.

Participation and preferences: If at all feasible, include the senior in meal preparation. Take into account their tastes and favorite recipes while maintaining nutritional balance.

Adapt to Preferences: Because of taste changes or dental difficulties, seniors may have special nutritional preferences. Adapt dishes to their preferences while keeping nutritional value in mind.

Hydration: Drink plenty of water throughout the day. Encourage the consumption of water and hydrating meals such as soups, fruits, and vegetables.

Healthy Snacks: Keep healthy snack alternatives on hand. Nuts, fruits, yogurt, and whole-grain crackers can all be used as healthy snacks in between meals.

Caregiver Assistance: Open communication is vital between caregivers and the elderly. Discuss food preferences, appetite fluctuations, and any issues with eating or preparing meals.

Routine and schedule: Establish a mealtime plan to maintain consistent and regular eating habits.

30 Day Alzheimer's Meal Plan for seniors

Day 1:

- **Breakfast:** Blueberry Spinach Smoothie

- **Lunch:** Salmon Salad

- **Dinner:** Salmon with Turmeric and Vegetables

- **Snacks:** Turmeric Roasted Chickpeas

- **Dessert:** Turmeric Ginger Tea

Day 2:

- **Breakfast:** Salmon and Avocado Toast

- **Lunch:** Mediterranean Chickpea Salad

- **Dinner:** Quinoa and Vegetable Stir-Fry

- **Snacks:** Berry and Greek Yogurt Parfait

- **Dessert:** Green Tea Berry Infusion

Day 3:

- **Breakfast:** Turmeric Oatmeal

- **Lunch:** Spinach and Berry Salad

- **Dinner:** Sweet Potato and Spinach Curry

- **Snacks:** Apple Peanut Butter Sandwiches

- **Dessert:** Beetroot Carrot Juice

Day 4:

- **Breakfast:** Egg and Veggie Scramble

- **Lunch:** Tuna Avocado Wrap

- **Dinner:** Turkey and Vegetable Skewers

- **Snacks:** Cottage Cheese and Pineapple Delight

- **Dessert:** Walnut Date Shake

Day 5:

- **Breakfast:** Quinoa Breakfast Bowl

- **Lunch:** Bowl of Sweet Potatoes with Black Beans

- **Dinner:** Baked Cod with Lemon and Herbs

- **Snacks:** Spinach and Feta Stuffed Mushrooms

- **Dessert:** Spinach and Pineapple Green Juice

Day 6:

- **Breakfast:** Chia Seed Pudding

- **Lunch:** Broccoli and Cheddar Soup

- **Dinner:** Eggplant and Chickpea Curry

- **Snacks:** Hummus and Veggie Sticks

- **Dessert:** Almond Butter Protein Shake

Day 7:

- **Breakfast:** Whole Grain Pancakes with Berries

- **Lunch:** Grilled Chicken and Veggie Skewers

- **Dinner:** Mediterranean Chicken and Vegetable Skillet

- **Snacks:** Coconut-Curry Popcorn

- **Dessert:** Matcha Green Tea Latte

Day 8:

- **Breakfast:** Greek Yogurt Parfait

- **Lunch:** Tomato Basil Mozzarella Salad

- **Dinner:** Baked Butternut Squash Risotto

- **Snacks:** Kale Chips

- **Dessert:** Walnut Date Shake

Day 9:

- **Breakfast:** Spinach and Mushroom Omelet

- **Lunch:** Chicken and Vegetable Brown Rice Bowl

- **Dinner:** Herb-Roasted Turkey Breast with Vegetables

- **Snacks:** Cinnamon-Roasted Almonds

- **Dessert:** Spinach and Pineapple Green Juice

Day 10:

- **Breakfast:** Coconut-Berry Smoothie Bowl

- **Lunch:** Bean and Spinach Quesadilla

- **Dinner:** Chickpea and Spinach Coconut Curry

- **Snacks:** Hummus and Veggie Sticks

- **Dessert:** Almond Butter Protein Shake

Day 11:

- **Breakfast:** Blueberry Spinach Smoothie

- **Lunch:** Bowl of Sweet Potatoes with Black Beans

- **Dinner:** Salmon with Turmeric and Vegetables

- **Snacks:** Cottage Cheese and Pineapple Delight

- **Dessert:** Matcha Green Tea Latte

Day 12:

- **Breakfast:** Salmon and Avocado Toast

- **Lunch:** Broccoli and Cheddar Soup

- **Dinner:** Quinoa and Vegetable Stir-Fry

- **Snacks:** Spinach and Feta Stuffed Mushrooms

- **Dessert:** Cocoa Banana Almond Milkshake

Day 13:

- **Breakfast:** Turmeric Oatmeal

- **Lunch:** Grilled Chicken and Veggie Skewers

- **Dinner:** Eggplant and Chickpea Curry

- **Snacks:** Coconut-Curry Popcorn

- **Dessert:** Pomegranate Berry Juice

Day 14:

- **Breakfast:** Egg and Veggie Scramble

- **Lunch:** Mediterranean Chickpea Salad

- **Dinner:** Turkey and Vegetable Skewers

- **Snacks:** Berry and Greek Yogurt Parfait

- **Dessert:** Green Tea Berry Infusion

Day 15:

- **Breakfast:** Turmeric Oatmeal

- **Lunch:** Tuna Avocado Wrap

- **Dinner:** Quinoa and Vegetable Stir-Fry

- **Snacks:** Hummus and Veggie Sticks

- **Dessert:** Walnut Date Shake

Day 16:

- **Breakfast:** Quinoa Breakfast Bowl

- **Lunch:** Spinach and Berry Salad

- **Dinner:** Sweet Potato and Spinach Curry

- **Snacks:** Apple Peanut Butter Sandwiches

- **Dessert:** Beetroot Carrot Juice

Day 17:

- **Breakfast:** Chia Seed Pudding

- **Lunch:** Tuna Avocado Wrap

- **Dinner:** Baked Cod with Lemon and Herbs

- **Snacks:** Kale Chips

- **Dessert:** Walnut Date Shake

Day 18:

- **Breakfast:** Whole Grain Pancakes with Berries

- **Lunch:** Bowl of Sweet Potatoes with Black Beans

- **Dinner:** Eggplant and Chickpea Curry

- **Snacks:** Spinach and Feta Stuffed Mushrooms

- **Dessert:** Spinach and Pineapple Green Juice

Day 19:

- **Breakfast:** Coconut-Berry Smoothie Bowl

- **Lunch:** Bean and Spinach Quesadilla

- **Dinner:** Chickpea and Spinach Coconut Curry

- **Snacks:** Hummus and Veggie Sticks

- **Dessert:** Almond Butter Protein Shake

Day 20:

- **Breakfast:** Blueberry Spinach Smoothie

- **Lunch:** Bowl of Sweet Potatoes with Black Beans

- **Dinner:** Salmon with Turmeric and Vegetables

- **Snacks:** Cottage Cheese and Pineapple Delight

- **Dessert:** Matcha Green Tea Latte

Day 21:

- **Breakfast:** Salmon and Avocado Toast

- **Lunch:** Broccoli and Cheddar Soup

- **Dinner:** Quinoa and Vegetable Stir-Fry

- **Snacks:** Spinach and Feta Stuffed Mushrooms

- **Dessert:** Cocoa Banana Almond Milkshake

Day 22:

- **Breakfast:** Turmeric Oatmeal

- **Lunch:** Grilled Chicken and Veggie Skewers

- **Dinner:** Eggplant and Chickpea Curry

- **Snacks:** Coconut-Curry Popcorn

- **Dessert:** Pomegranate Berry Juice

Day 23:

- **Breakfast:** Greek Yogurt Parfait

- **Lunch:** Tomato Basil Mozzarella Salad

- **Dinner:** Baked Butternut Squash Risotto

- **Snacks:** Kale Chips

- **Dessert:** Walnut Date Shake

Day 24:

- **Breakfast:** Spinach and Mushroom Omelet

- **Lunch:** Chicken and Vegetable Brown Rice Bowl

- **Dinner:** Herb-Roasted Turkey Breast with Vegetables

- **Snacks:** Cinnamon-Roasted Almonds

- **Dessert:** Spinach and Pineapple Green Juice

Day 25:

- **Breakfast:** Coconut-Berry Smoothie Bowl

- **Lunch:** Bean and Spinach Quesadilla

- **Dinner:** Chickpea and Spinach Coconut Curry

- **Snacks:** Hummus and Veggie Sticks

- **Dessert:** Almond Butter Protein Shake

Day 26:

- **Breakfast:** Blueberry Spinach Smoothie

- **Lunch:** Bowl of Sweet Potatoes with Black Beans

- **Dinner:** Salmon with Turmeric and Vegetables

- **Snacks:** Cottage Cheese and Pineapple Delight

- **Dessert:** Matcha Green Tea Latte

Day 27:

- **Breakfast:** Salmon and Avocado Toast

- **Lunch:** Broccoli and Cheddar Soup

- **Dinner:** Quinoa and Vegetable Stir-Fry

- **Snacks:** Spinach and Feta Stuffed Mushrooms

- **Dessert:** Cocoa Banana Almond Milkshake

Day 28:

- **Breakfast:** Turmeric Oatmeal

- **Lunch:** Grilled Chicken and Veggie Skewers

- **Dinner:** Eggplant and Chickpea Curry

- **Snacks:** Coconut-Curry Popcorn

- **Dessert:** Pomegranate Berry Juice

Day 29:

- **Breakfast:** Greek Yogurt Parfait

- **Lunch:** Tomato Basil Mozzarella Salad

- **Dinner:** Baked Butternut Squash Risotto

- **Snacks:** Kale Chips

- **Dessert:** Walnut Date Shake

Day 30:

- **Breakfast:** Spinach and Mushroom Omelet

- **Lunch:** Chicken and Vegetable Brown Rice Bowl

- **Dinner:** Herb-Roasted Turkey Breast with Vegetables

- **Snacks:** Cinnamon-Roasted Almonds

- **Dessert:** Spinach and Pineapple Green Juice

Chapter 4: Breakfasts Recipes for Boosting Brain Function

Blueberry Spinach Smoothie

Ingredients:

- 1 cup fresh spinach

- 1/2 cup blueberries (fresh or frozen)

- 1/2 banana

- 1/2 cup Greek yogurt

- 1 tablespoon chia seeds

- 1/2 cup almond milk

Instructions:

1. Blend spinach, blueberries, banana, Greek yogurt, chia seeds, and almond milk until smooth.

2. Pour into a glass and serve immediately.

Preparation Time: 5 minutes

Nutritional Value: Rich in antioxidants, vitamins, minerals, and healthy fats from chia seeds.

Salmon and Avocado Toast

Ingredients:

- 2 slices whole-grain bread

- 1/2 avocado, mashed

- Smoked salmon

- Lemon juice

- Fresh dill (optional)

Instructions:

1. Toast the bread slices.

2. Spread mashed avocado on the toast.

3. Top with smoked salmon.

4. Squeeze fresh lemon juice on top and garnish with dill, if desired.

Preparation Time: 10 minutes

Nutritional Value: Provides omega-3 fatty acids from salmon, healthy fats from avocado, and whole grains.

Turmeric Oatmeal

Ingredients:

- 1 cup rolled oats

- 2 cups of water or preferred milk

- 1/2 teaspoon ground turmeric

- 1/2 teaspoon cinnamon

- Chopped nuts (walnuts, almonds) and berries for topping

Instructions:

1. Cook oats in water or milk according to package instructions.

2. Stir in turmeric and cinnamon while cooking.

3. Serve topped with chopped nuts and berries.

Preparation Time: 15 minutes

Nutritional Value: Contains fiber from oats, anti-inflammatory properties from turmeric, and antioxidants from nuts and berries.

Egg and Veggie Scramble

Ingredients:

- 2 eggs

- Chopped vegetables (bell peppers, spinach, tomatoes)

- Olive oil

- Herbs (thyme, basil)

- Salt and pepper to taste

Instructions:

1. Heat olive oil in a pan and sauté chopped vegetables until tender.

2. Whisk eggs in a bowl and pour into the pan with vegetables.

3. Cook until eggs are scrambled and fully cooked.

4. Season with herbs, salt, and pepper.

Preparation Time: 10 minutes

Nutritional Value: High in protein from eggs, vitamins, and antioxidants from vegetables.

Quinoa Breakfast Bowl

Ingredients:

- 1/2 cup cooked quinoa

- Greek yogurt

- Mixed berries

- Honey or maple syrup

- Chopped nuts (almonds, pecans)

Instructions:

1. Place cooked quinoa in a bowl.

2. Top with Greek yogurt, mixed berries, drizzle with honey or maple syrup, and sprinkle with chopped nuts.

Preparation Time: 5 minutes

Nutritional Value: Contains protein and fiber from quinoa, probiotics from Greek yogurt, antioxidants from berries, and healthy fats from nuts.

Chia Seed Pudding

Ingredients:

- 3 tablespoons chia seeds
- 1 cup almond milk
- 1/2 teaspoon vanilla extract
- Sliced bananas or berries for topping

Instructions:

1. Mix chia seeds, almond milk, and vanilla extract in a bowl. Stir well.

2. Refrigerate for at least 2 hours or overnight until it thickens.

3. Serve topped with sliced bananas or berries.

Preparation Time: 5 minutes (+ refrigeration time)

Nutritional Value: High in omega-3 fatty acids, fiber, and antioxidants from chia seeds and fruits.

Whole Grain Pancakes with Berries

Ingredients:

- 1 cup whole wheat flour
- 1 tablespoon baking powder
- 1 tablespoon honey or maple syrup
- 1 cup milk of choice
- Mixed berries for topping

Instructions:

1. In a bowl, mix whole wheat flour, baking powder, honey or maple syrup, and milk to form a batter.

2. Heat a non-stick pan and pour batter to make pancakes.

3. Serve topped with mixed berries.

Preparation Time: 20 minutes

Nutritional Value: Provides whole grains, fiber, and antioxidants from berries.

Greek Yogurt Parfait

Ingredients:

- Greek yogurt

- Granola

- Sliced bananas or berries

- Honey or maple syrup (optional)

Instructions:

1. Layer Greek yogurt, granola, and sliced bananas or berries in a glass or bowl.

2. Drizzle with honey or maple syrup if desired.

Preparation Time: 5 minutes

Nutritional Value: Contains probiotics from Greek yogurt, fiber from granola, and antioxidants from fruits.

Spinach and Mushroom Omelet

Ingredients:

- 2 eggs

- Handful of spinach

- Sliced mushrooms

- Grated cheese (optional)

- Olive oil

- Salt and pepper to taste

Instructions:

1. In a bowl, beat eggs and add salt and pepper to taste.

2. Heat olive oil in a pan and sauté spinach and mushrooms until tender.

3. Pour beaten eggs into the pan and cook until set.

4. Sprinkle with grated cheese if desired and fold the omelet.

Preparation Time: 10 minutes

Nutritional Value: High in protein from eggs, vitamins, and minerals from spinach and mushrooms.

Coconut-Berry Smoothie Bowl

Ingredients:

- 1 cup mixed berries (frozen or fresh)

- 1/2 cup coconut milk

- 1/4 cup Greek yogurt

- Garnishes: sliced almonds, shredded coconut, and chia seeds

Instructions:

1. Blend mixed berries, coconut milk, and Greek yogurt until smooth.

2. Pour into a bowl and garnish with preferred toppings.

Preparation Time: 5 minutes

Nutritional Value: Provides antioxidants, healthy fats, and probiotics from coconut milk and yogurt, as well as fiber and omega-3s from berries and nuts.

Chapter 5: Lunches Recipes to Enhance Cognitive Abilities

Salmon Salad

Ingredients:

- 2 cups mixed greens

- 1/2 cup cooked salmon (grilled or baked)

- 1/4 cup cherry tomatoes

- 1/4 cup cucumber slices

- 1 tablespoon olive oil

- 1 tablespoon lemon juice

- Salt and pepper to taste

Instructions:

1. Toss mixed greens, cherry tomatoes, and cucumber in a bowl.

2. Top with cooked salmon.

3. Pour in some lemon juice and olive oil.

4. Season with salt and pepper.

Nutritional Value: Omega-3 fatty acids from salmon support brain health, Antioxidants from mixed greens, tomatoes, and cucumber.

Preparation time: 15 minutes.

Mediterranean Chickpea Salad

Ingredients:

- 1 can chickpeas, drained and rinsed
- 1/2 cup cherry tomatoes, halved
- 1/4 cup diced red onion
- 1/4 cup chopped cucumber
- 2 tablespoons chopped fresh parsley
- 2 tablespoons olive oil
- 1 tablespoon lemon juice
- Salt and pepper to taste

Instructions:

1. Combine chickpeas, cherry tomatoes, red onion, cucumber, and parsley in a bowl.

2. Drizzle with olive oil and lemon juice, season with salt and pepper.

Nutritional Value: Chickpeas are rich in folate and protein. Olive oil provides healthy fats.

Preparation time: 10 minutes.

Spinach and Berry Salad

Ingredients:

- 2 cups fresh spinach leaves

- 1/2 cup mixed berries (blueberries, strawberries)

- 1/4 cup sliced almonds

- 2 tablespoons balsamic vinaigrette

Instructions:

1. Toss spinach leaves, mixed berries, and sliced almonds in a bowl.

2. Drizzle with balsamic vinaigrette.

Nutritional Value: Spinach provides iron and antioxidants. Berries offer antioxidants and vitamins.

Preparation time: 10 minutes.

Tuna Avocado Wrap

Ingredients:

- 1 can tuna, drained

- 1 ripe avocado, mashed

- 2 whole-grain tortillas

- 1/2 cup shredded lettuce

- 1/4 cup diced tomatoes

Instructions:

1. Mix tuna and mashed avocado in a bowl.

2. Spread the mixture on whole-grain tortillas.

3. Top with shredded lettuce and diced tomatoes, roll into wraps.

Nutritional Value: Omega-3s from tuna support brain health. Avocado provides healthy fats.

Preparation time: 10 minutes.

Bowl of Sweet Potatoes with Black Beans

Ingredients:

- 1 cup cooked black beans
- 1 medium sweet potato, diced and roasted
- 1/4 cup diced red bell pepper
- 2 tablespoons chopped cilantro
- 1 tablespoon olive oil
- 1 tablespoon lime juice

Instructions:

1. Combine black beans, roasted sweet potato, diced bell pepper, and cilantro in a bowl.

2. Drizzle with olive oil and lime juice, toss gently.

Nutritional Value: Sweet potatoes offer antioxidants and vitamins. Black beans provide fiber and protein.

Preparation time: 25 minutes.

Broccoli and Cheddar Soup

Ingredients:

- 2 cups chopped broccoli

- 1 cup vegetable or chicken broth

- 1/2 cup shredded cheddar cheese

- 1/4 cup diced onions

- 1 clove garlic, minced

- Salt and pepper to taste

Instructions:

1. In a pot, sauté onions and garlic until fragrant.

2. Add chopped broccoli and broth, simmer until broccoli is tender.

3. Blend the mixture until smooth, return to the pot.

4. Stir in the shredded cheddar cheese until completely melted.

Nutritional Value: Broccoli is high in antioxidants and vitamins. Cheddar cheese provides calcium and protein.

Preparation time: 30 minutes.

Grilled Chicken and Veggie Skewers

Ingredients:

- 1 chicken breast, cut into chunks

- Assorted vegetables (bell peppers, zucchini, mushrooms)

- 1 tablespoon olive oil

- 1 teaspoon dried herbs (rosemary, thyme)

- Salt and pepper to taste

Instructions:

1. Thread chicken chunks and vegetables onto skewers.

2. Mix olive oil, dried herbs, salt, and pepper.

3. Brush the skewers with the mixture.

4. Grill until chicken is cooked through.

Nutritional Value: Chicken provides protein. Vegetables offer vitamins and antioxidants.

Preparation time: 25 minutes.

Tomato Basil Mozzarella Salad

Ingredients:

- 1 cup cherry tomatoes, halved
- 1/2 cup fresh mozzarella cheese, diced
- 1/4 cup fresh basil leaves, chopped
- 2 tablespoons balsamic vinegar
- 1 tablespoon olive oil
- Salt and pepper to taste

Instructions:

1. Combine cherry tomatoes, mozzarella, and chopped basil in a bowl.

2. Sprinkle with olive oil and balsamic vinegar.

3. Season with salt and pepper.

Nutritional Value: Tomatoes contain antioxidants and vitamin C. Mozzarella provides calcium and protein.

Preparation time: 10 minutes.

Chicken and Vegetable Brown Rice Bowl

Ingredients:

- 1 cup cooked brown rice

- 1 grilled chicken breast, sliced

- 1/2 cup steamed broccoli florets

- 1/4 cup sliced carrots

- 2 tablespoons soy sauce

- 1 tablespoon sesame oil

- 1 teaspoon grated ginger

Instructions:

1. Arrange cooked brown rice in a bowl.

2. Top with sliced grilled chicken, steamed broccoli, and sliced carrots.

3. Mix soy sauce, sesame oil, and grated ginger, drizzle over the bowl.

Nutritional Value: Brown rice provides fiber and complex carbs. Chicken provides protein. Vegetables offer vitamins and antioxidants.

Preparation time: 25 minutes.

Bean and Spinach Quesadilla

Ingredients:

- 2 whole-grain tortillas

- 1/2 cup canned black beans (drained and rinsed)

- 1 cup fresh spinach leaves

- 1/2 cup shredded cheddar cheese

- 1 tablespoon olive oil

Instructions:

1. Heat olive oil in a pan, place one tortilla in the pan.

2. Spread black beans, spinach, and shredded cheddar on the tortilla.

3. Cover with the second tortilla, press gently, and cook until golden.

4. Flip and cook the other side until cheese melts.

5. Cut into wedges and serve.

Nutritional Value: Black beans offer fiber and protein. Spinach provides iron and antioxidants. Whole-grain tortillas offer complex carbohydrates.

Preparation time: 15 minutes.

Chapter 6: Dinners Recipes for Supporting Brain Health

Salmon with Turmeric and Vegetables

Ingredients:

- 2 salmon fillets

- 1 teaspoon turmeric

- Assorted vegetables (broccoli, bell peppers, carrots)

- Olive oil

- Salt and pepper

Instructions:

1. Preheat oven to 375°F (190°C).

2. Rub turmeric, salt, and pepper on salmon fillets.

3. Place salmon on a baking sheet, surrounded by assorted vegetables tossed in olive oil.

4. Bake for 15-20 minutes or until salmon is cooked through.

Preparation Time: 25 minutes

Nutritional Value: Omega-3 fatty acids from salmon for brain health Antioxidants from vegetables, especially turmeric, for reducing inflammation

Quinoa and Vegetable Stir-Fry

Ingredients:

- 1 cup quinoa

- Assorted vegetables (bell peppers, spinach, mushrooms)

- Garlic cloves (minced)

- Olive oil

- Soy sauce

Instructions:

1. Cook quinoa according to package instructions.

2. In a pan, sauté minced garlic in olive oil.

3. Add chopped vegetables and cook until tender.

4. Add cooked quinoa and soy sauce, stir-frying until combined.

Preparation Time: 30 minutes

Nutritional Value: Quinoa for complex carbohydrates and protein. Vegetables for antioxidants and vitamins. Healthy fats from olive oil for brain health.

Sweet Potato and Spinach Curry

Ingredients:

- Sweet potatoes (diced)

- Spinach leaves

- Onion (chopped)

- Curry paste

- Coconut milk

- Olive oil

Instructions:

1. In a pot, sauté chopped onion in olive oil until soft.

2. Add diced sweet potatoes and cook until slightly tender.

3. Stir in curry paste, then add coconut milk and simmer.

4. Add spinach leaves, cooking until wilted.

Preparation Time: 40 minutes

Nutritional Value: Sweet potatoes for complex carbohydrates. Spinach for antioxidants and vitamins, Healthy fats from coconut milk

Turkey and Vegetable Skewers

Ingredients:

- Turkey breast (cubed)

- Bell peppers (sliced)

- Red onion (sliced)

- Olive oil

- Italian seasoning

- Garlic powder

Instructions:

1. Preheat the grill or oven to medium-high.

2. Thread turkey cubes, bell peppers, and onion slices onto skewers.

3. Brush skewers with olive oil and sprinkle with Italian seasoning and garlic powder.

4. Grill or bake for 10-15 minutes until turkey is cooked through.

Preparation Time: 25 minutes

Nutritional Value: Lean protein from turkey, Antioxidants from bell peppers and onion, Healthy fats from olive oil

Baked Cod with Lemon and Herbs

Ingredients:

- Cod fillets

- Lemon

- Fresh herbs (rosemary, thyme)

- Garlic (minced)

- Olive oil

- Salt and pepper

Instructions:

1. Preheat oven to 400°F (200°C).

2. Place cod fillets on a baking sheet lined with foil.

3. Drizzle with olive oil, sprinkle minced garlic, fresh herbs, and lemon juice.

4. Season with salt and pepper, then bake for 15-20 minutes.

Preparation Time: 25 minutes

Nutritional Value: Omega-3s from cod for brain health, Antioxidants from fresh herbs and lemon

Eggplant and Chickpea Curry

Ingredients:

- Eggplant (cubed)

- Chickpeas (cooked)

- Tomato sauce

- Onion (chopped)

- Garlic (minced)

- Curry powder

- Coconut oil

Instructions:

1. In a pan, sauté chopped onion and minced garlic in coconut oil.

2. Add cubed eggplant and cook until slightly soft.

3. Stir in chickpeas, tomato sauce, and curry powder.

4. Simmer for 15-20 minutes until flavors blend.

Preparation Time: 35 minutes

Nutritional Value: Eggplant for fiber and antioxidants, Chickpeas for protein and complex carbohydrates, Healthy fats from coconut oil

Mediterranean Chicken and Vegetable Skillet

Ingredients:

- Chicken thighs (boneless, skinless)
- Zucchini (sliced)
- Cherry tomatoes
- Kalamata olives (pitted)
- Olive oil
- Garlic (minced)
- Oregano (dried)
- Salt and pepper

Instructions:

1. Add dried oregano, salt, and pepper to chicken thighs for seasoning.

2. In a skillet, cook chicken in olive oil until browned and cooked through. Remove and set aside.

3. In the same skillet, sauté minced garlic, add zucchini, tomatoes, and olives. Cook until vegetables are tender.

4. Add chicken back to the skillet, warm through, and serve.

Preparation Time: 30 minutes

Nutritional Value: Protein from chicken, Olives and olive oil provide healthy fats, Antioxidants from tomatoes and zucchini

Baked Butternut Squash Risotto

Ingredients:

- Arborio rice

- Butternut squash (cubed)

- Onion (chopped)

- Vegetable broth

- Parmesan cheese

- Sage leaves

- Olive oil

- Black pepper

Instructions:

1. In olive oil, sauté chopped onion until translucent.

2. Add Arborio rice and cubed butternut squash, stirring for a few minutes.

3. Gradually add vegetable broth while stirring occasionally until the rice is cooked.

4. Stir in grated Parmesan cheese, chopped sage leaves, and black pepper before serving.

Preparation Time: 40 minutes

Nutritional Value: Complex carbohydrates from Arborio rice, Vitamins and fiber from butternut squash, Protein and calcium from Parmesan cheese

Herb-Roasted Turkey Breast with Vegetables

Ingredients:

- Turkey breast (boneless)

- Potatoes (cut into chunks)

- Carrots (sliced)

- Rosemary (fresh)

- Thyme (fresh)

- Garlic powder

- Olive oil

- Salt and pepper

Instructions:

1. Preheat oven to 375°F (190°C).

2. Rub turkey breast with olive oil, garlic powder, fresh rosemary, and thyme.

3. Place turkey in a baking dish surrounded by potatoes and carrots.

4. Roast for about 1 hour or until turkey is cooked through and vegetables are tender.

Preparation Time: 1 hour 15 minutes

Nutritional Value: Lean protein from turkey, Potatoes and carrots provide vitamins and minerals. Antioxidants and flavor from fresh herbs

Chickpea and Spinach Coconut Curry

Ingredients:

- Chickpeas (canned)

- Spinach leaves

- Coconut milk

- Onion (chopped)

- Curry powder

- Ginger (minced)

- Turmeric powder

- Olive oil

- Basmati rice (optional)

Instructions:

1. In a pan, sauté chopped onion and minced ginger in olive oil.

2. Add drained chickpeas, curry powder, and turmeric powder. Cook for a few minutes.

3. Stir in coconut milk and simmer until chickpeas are heated through.

4. Add spinach leaves and cook until wilted. Serve with rice if desired.

Preparation Time: 30 minutes

Nutritional Value: Protein and fiber from chickpeas, Iron and vitamins from spinach, Healthy fats from coconut milk

Broccoli and Walnut Pasta

Ingredients:

- Whole wheat pasta

- Broccoli florets

- Walnuts (chopped)

- Garlic (minced)

- Olive oil

- Lemon zest

- Red pepper flakes

- Parmesan cheese (optional)

Instructions:

1. Cook whole wheat pasta according to package instructions.

2. In a pan, sauté minced garlic in olive oil until fragrant.

3. Add broccoli florets, chopped walnuts, lemon zest, and red pepper flakes. Cook until broccoli is tender.

4. Toss cooked pasta with the broccoli mixture. Add grated Parmesan cheese if desired before serving.

Preparation Time: 25 minutes

Nutritional Value: Whole wheat pasta for complex carbohydrates, Vitamins and fiber from broccoli

Omega-3s from walnuts

Chapter 7: Recipes for Nourishing and Delicious Brain-Boosting Snacks

Berry and Greek Yogurt Parfait

Ingredients:

- 1 cup Greek yogurt

- 1/2 cup berries (blueberries, strawberries, raspberries)

- 1 tablespoon honey or maple syrup

- Granola (optional)

Instructions:

1. In a bowl or glass, layer Greek yogurt, mixed berries, and a drizzle of honey or maple syrup.

2. Optionally, top with granola for added crunch.

3. Serve immediately.

Preparation Time: 5 minutes

Nutritional Value: Greek yogurt provides protein and probiotics while berries offer antioxidants and vitamins.

Turmeric Roasted Chickpeas

Ingredients:

- 1 can chickpeas (15 oz), drained and rinsed

- 1 tablespoon olive oil

- 1 teaspoon turmeric

- 1/2 teaspoon cumin

- Salt to taste

Instructions:

1. Preheat oven to 400°F (200°C).

2. Using a paper towel, pat dry the chickpeas.

3. In a bowl, toss chickpeas with olive oil, turmeric, cumin, and salt.

4. Spread the chickpeas on a baking sheet and bake for 20-25 minutes until crispy.

Preparation Time: 30 minutes (including baking) **Nutritional Value:** Chickpeas offer fiber and protein, while turmeric has anti-inflammatory properties.

Apple Peanut Butter Sandwiches

Ingredients:

- 1 apple, sliced into rounds

- Peanut butter (or almond butter)

- Granola or chopped nuts (optional)

Instructions:

1. Spread peanut butter on one apple slice and top with another slice to make a sandwich.

2. Optionally, roll the edges in granola or chopped nuts for added crunch.

Preparation Time: 5 minutes

Nutritional Value: Apples offer fiber and antioxidants while peanut butter provides healthy fats and protein.

Cottage Cheese and Pineapple Delight

Ingredients:

- Cottage cheese

- Fresh pineapple chunks

Instructions:

1. Serve cottage cheese topped with fresh pineapple chunks.

Preparation Time: 5 minutes
Nutritional Value: Cottage cheese provides protein and calcium, while pineapple offers vitamins and antioxidants.

Spinach and Feta Stuffed Mushrooms

Ingredients:

- Large mushrooms, stems removed

- Spinach, chopped

- Feta cheese

- Garlic, minced

- Olive oil

- Salt and pepper to taste

Instructions:

1. Preheat oven to 375°F (190°C).

2. In a pan, sauté spinach and garlic in olive oil until wilted. Mix in crumbled feta cheese.

3. Stuff the mushroom caps with the spinach and feta mixture.

4. Bake for 15-20 minutes until mushrooms are tender.

Preparation Time: 30 minutes (including baking) **Nutritional Value:** Spinach is rich in antioxidants and mushrooms offer various vitamins and minerals.

Hummus and Veggie Sticks

Ingredients:

- Homemade or store-bought hummus

- Vegetable sticks (carrots, cucumber, and bell peppers)

Instructions:

1. Wash and cut vegetables into sticks.

2. Serve with hummus as a dip.

Preparation Time: 10 minutes (if using store-bought hummus)
Nutritional Value: Vegetables offer vitamins and antioxidants, while hummus provides protein and healthy fats.

Coconut-Curry Popcorn

Ingredients:

- Popped popcorn (plain, air-popped)

- 2 tablespoons coconut oil

- 1 teaspoon curry powder

- Salt to taste

Instructions:

1. In a small pan, melt coconut oil over low heat.

2. Stir in curry powder and mix well.

3. Drizzle the coconut-curry mixture over the popped popcorn.

4. Sprinkle with salt and toss to coat evenly.

Preparation Time: 10 minutes

Nutritional Value: Popcorn is a whole grain and coconut oil offers medium-chain triglycerides that may benefit brain health.

Kale Chips

Ingredients:

- Fresh kale leaves, washed and dried

- Olive oil

- Salt or seasoning of choice (paprika, garlic powder)

Instructions:

1. Preheat oven to 300°F (150°C).

2. Tear kale into bite-sized pieces and place on a baking sheet.

3. Drizzle with olive oil and sprinkle with seasoning.

4. Bake for 10-15 minutes until crisp.

Preparation Time: 20 minutes (including baking)

Nutritional Value: Kale is rich in antioxidants and vitamins, providing essential nutrients for brain health.

Cinnamon-Roasted Almonds

Ingredients:

- 1 cup raw almonds

- one tablespoon melted coconut oil or olive oil

- 1 tablespoon maple syrup

- 1 teaspoon ground cinnamon

- Pinch of salt

Instructions:

1. Preheat oven to 300°F (150°C).

2. Mix almonds with melted oil, maple syrup, cinnamon, and salt.

3. Place on a baking sheet lined with parchment paper.

4. Bake for 20-25 minutes, stirring occasionally, until golden and fragrant.

Preparation Time: 30 minutes (including baking)

Nutritional Value: Almonds provide healthy fats and antioxidants, while cinnamon may have anti-inflammatory properties.

Chapter 8: Recipes for Brain-Boosting Beverages and Drinks

Turmeric Ginger Tea

Ingredients:

- 2 cups water
- 1 teaspoon turmeric powder or grated fresh turmeric
- 1 teaspoon grated ginger
- Honey (optional)

Instructions:

1. Boil water with turmeric and ginger for 10 minutes.
2. Strain and add honey if desired.
3. Serve hot.

Nutritional Value: Turmeric: provides curcumin, known for its anti-inflammatory properties. Ginger: Anti-inflammatory and antioxidant effects.

Green Tea Berry Infusion

Ingredients:

- 2 green tea bags

- 2 cups hot water

- 1/2 cup mixed berries (blueberries, strawberries)

Instructions:

1. Steep green tea bags in hot water for 3-5 minutes.

2. Add mixed berries and let it cool.

3. Refrigerate and serve cold over ice.

Nutritional Value: Green tea: Contains antioxidants like catechins, Berries: antioxidants and vitamin C.

Beetroot Carrot Juice

Ingredients:

- 2 medium beetroots, peeled and chopped

- 3 carrots, peeled and chopped

- 1 apple, chopped

- 1-inch ginger (optional)

Instructions:

1. Juice all ingredients in a juicer.

2. Strain if needed and serve immediately.

Nutritional Value: Beetroots: High in nitrates and antioxidants, Carrots: Rich in beta-carotene and vitamins.

Walnut Date Shake

Ingredients:

- 1/2 cup walnuts

- 3-4 pitted dates

- 1 ripe banana

- 1 cup almond milk

- Cinnamon (optional)

Instructions:

1. Blend all ingredients until smooth.

2. Sprinkle cinnamon on top if desired.

3. Serve chilled.

Nutritional Value: Walnuts: Omega-3 fatty acids and antioxidants. Dates: Natural sweetener and fiber.

Spinach and Pineapple Green Juice

Ingredients:

- 2 cups fresh spinach leaves

- 1 cup chopped pineapple

- 1 cucumber, chopped

- 1 lemon, juiced

Instructions:

1. Juice spinach, pineapple, and cucumber.

2. Mix in lemon juice and serve over ice.

Nutritional Value: Spinach: vitamins A, C, K, and folate. Pineapple: Contains bromelain and antioxidants.

Almond Butter Protein Shake

Ingredients:

- 2 tablespoons almond butter

- 1 ripe banana

- 1 cup Greek yogurt

- 1/2 cup almond milk

- 1 tablespoon honey or maple syrup

- Ice cubes

Instructions:

1. Blend all ingredients until creamy.

2. Add ice cubes for desired thickness.

3. Pour into glasses and serve.

Nutritional Value: Almond butter: Healthy fats, vitamin E, and protein. Greek yogurt: Protein and probiotics.

Matcha Green Tea Latte

Ingredients:

- 1 teaspoon matcha powder

- 1 tablespoon hot water

- 1 cup almond milk

- Honey or maple syrup (optional)

Instructions:

1. Whisk matcha powder and hot water until smooth.

2. Heat almond milk in a saucepan until warm.

3. Pour milk into a cup and stir in the matcha mixture.

4. If desired, sweeten with honey or maple syrup.

Nutritional Value: Matcha: Contains antioxidants, including EGCG. Almond milk: Source of vitamin E and healthy fats.

Citrus Ginger Infused Water

Ingredients:

- 1 lemon, sliced

- 1 lime, sliced

- 1-inch fresh ginger, thinly sliced

- Fresh mint leaves

- 2 liters water (filtered or sparkling)

Instructions:

1. Add lemon, lime, ginger, and mint to a pitcher.

2. Fill the pitcher with water.

3. Refrigerate for a few hours to infuse flavors.

Nutritional Value: Citrus fruits: High in vitamin C and antioxidants. Ginger: Anti-inflammatory and digestive benefits.

Cocoa Banana Almond Milkshake

Ingredients:

- 2 ripe bananas

- 2 tablespoons cocoa powder

- 1 cup almond milk

- 1 tablespoon almond butter

- Ice cubes

Instructions:

1. Blend bananas, cocoa powder, almond milk, and almond butter until smooth.

2. Add ice cubes and blend again until creamy.

3. Pour into glasses and serve immediately.

Nutritional Value: Bananas: Potassium and vitamins B6, C. Cocoa: Antioxidants and flavonoids.

Pomegranate Berry Juice

Ingredients:

- 1 cup pomegranate seeds (or 100% pomegranate juice)

- 1/2 cup mixed berries (strawberries, raspberries)

- 1/2 cup coconut water

- Fresh mint leaves for garnish

Instructions:

1. Blend pomegranate seeds, mixed berries, and coconut water until smooth.

2. Strain if desired and garnish with mint leaves.

3. Serve chilled.

Nutritional Value: Pomegranate: High in antioxidants and polyphenols. Berries: Antioxidants and vitamins.

Chapter 9: Lifestyle Tips for Holistic Brain Health

1. Physical Activity: Engage in aerobic workouts, weight training, and other activities that increase blood flow to the brain, which aids cognitive performance. Basic daily activities such as walking or gardening can improve brain function.

2. Mental Stimulation: Continuous learning is crucial. Use puzzles, games, reading, or learning a new skill or language to keep the brain busy. Creative activities help to activate different brain regions. Engage in creative activities such as painting, writing, or playing musical instruments.

3. Sleep Quality: Maintain a consistent sleep schedule. To maintain brain health and cognitive performance, aim for 7-9 hours of quality sleep every night. Create a pleasant sleeping environment, restrict screen time before bed, and develop a calming nighttime routine.

4. Stress Management: Mindfulness and meditation are great relaxation techniques to reduce stress and promote brain health. Time Management is also important. It will help you avoid chronic stress; efficiently manage your job and commitments.

5. Maintain Associations: Maintain relationships with friends, family, or community groups to support mental health. Stay socially engaged by participating in group activities, volunteering, or joining groups.

6. Seek Professional Help for Mental Health: Address mental health issues promptly, obtaining treatment or counseling as needed. Deep breathing, yoga, and mindfulness are all practices that can help reduce anxiety and boost brain health.

7. Brain Health Screenings: Schedule routine check-ups to monitor and manage health issues that may have an influence on brain health, such as diabetes, high blood pressure, or cholesterol.

8. Avoid bad habits: Excessive alcohol consumption can impair brain function; moderate consumption is recommended. Smoking causes blood vessel damage and increases the risk of cognitive loss.

9. Safety Precautions: Protective Equipment: When participating in sports or activities that are prone to head injuries, wear helmets and other protective gear. Reduce the danger of falling, especially for seniors, to avoid head injuries.

10. Brain Exercises: Participate in activities that are expressly meant to challenge and exercise the brain, such as brain-training apps or games.

11. Consistent Brain Rest: Provide appropriate pauses for the brain throughout work or study sessions to avoid mental weariness and burnout.

12. Environmental Factors: Reduce your exposure to pollutants, chemicals, and poisons that can affect your brain's health.

Social Engagement and Other Lifestyle Factors for

Social engagement is critical in the management of Alzheimer's disease, particularly for seniors, providing several cognitive, social, and psychological benefits:

Cognitive Stimulation: Participating in social activities improves memory, problem-solving abilities, and communication skills. Interaction with others exposes seniors to fresh ideas, viewpoints, and knowledge, promoting constant learning and brain health.

Emotional Health: Social interaction combats the feelings of loneliness and isolation that many seniors with Alzheimer's suffer, fostering a sense of belonging and togetherness.

Emotional Support: Being a part of a social circle gives emotional support, which reduces stress and improves general well-being.

Building Cognitive Reserve: Active social interaction contributes to the development of cognitive reserve, a buffer that may postpone or reduce the pace of cognitive impairment in Alzheimer's disease.

Physical Health Advantages: Socially active elders are more likely to embrace healthier lifestyles, such as frequent physical activity and improved food habits, which benefit overall health.

Practical Support: Social networks may comprise family, friends, or support organizations that provide elders and their caregivers with practical advice, resources, and help.

Alzheimer's Social Engagement Strategies:

Participate in activities intended expressly for people with Alzheimer's disease, such as art therapy, music programs, or memory-enhancing games.

Join Alzheimer's support groups: which provide a secure environment for sharing experiences, advice, and emotional support with others facing similar issues. Visits from family, friends, or volunteers on a regular basis provide companionship and social engagement.

Preventive Action: Because of its impact on cognitive stimulation and brain health, early social interaction may potentially lessen the likelihood or postpone the onset of Alzheimer's symptoms.

Adaptability: Ensure inclusion by adapting social activities to the changing needs and capacities of people with Alzheimer's.

Patience and Understanding: Promote understanding and acceptance of behavioral changes related to the condition by encouraging patience and empathy within social networks.

Caregiver Support Groups: Socialization for seniors with Alzheimer's disease frequently includes caregivers, highlighting the significance of support for them as well.

Conclusion

Embracing the journey toward Alzheimer's reversal and holistic well-being for seniors, this cookbook stands as a comprehensive guide merging culinary delights with scientific wisdom. Delving into the intricacies of Alzheimer's, it offers a multifaceted approach to nourishing the body and mind.

Through meticulously curated recipes, it champions the Alzheimer's Reversal Diet, emphasizing nutrient-rich ingredients tailored for cognitive support. From brain-boosting beverages to nutrient-dense meals, each recipe is a testament to the power of food in promoting brain health. The emphasis on essential ingredients, meal planning, and lifestyle adjustments creates a holistic foundation for combating cognitive decline.

Beyond recipes, this cookbook delves into the nuanced world of Alzheimer's, elucidating its types, symptoms, and preventive measures. It champions the role of social engagement, cognitive stimulation, and physical activity in managing Alzheimer's.

The book accentuates the importance of a balanced lifestyle, advocating for mental stimulation, quality sleep, stress management, and regular check-ups.

Recognizing the significance of social connections, it highlights the role of social engagement in Alzheimer's management, fostering emotional well-being and cognitive reserve for seniors. The inclusion of meal plans, lifestyle tips, and caregiver involvement ensures a comprehensive approach to support individuals navigating Alzheimer's.

Ultimately, this cookbook isn't merely a collection of recipes; it's a holistic roadmap toward Alzheimer's management. It's a compassionate companion for seniors and caregivers, offering guidance, empowerment, and hope in the journey toward improved brain health and quality of life.

In the pursuit of reversing the impact of Alzheimer's, this cookbook serves as a beacon of empowerment, merging nutrition, lifestyle adjustments, and emotional support into a transformative experience. It's a celebration of resilience, fostering a path toward cognitive well-being, one delicious recipe and supportive tip at a time.

Bonus: 15 Paged Seven-Day Meal Planner

SEVEN DAY MEAL
PLANNER

WEEK _______________

Monday
Tuesday
Wednesday
Thursday
Friday
Saturday
Sunday

To Do List

- ☐ _______________
- ☐ _______________
- ☐ _______________
- ☐ _______________
- ☐ _______________
- ☐ _______________
- ☐ _______________
- ☐ _______________
- ☐ _______________
- ☐ _______________
- ☐ _______________
- ☐ _______________

Notes

____

____

____

____

____

____

____

____

SEVEN DAY MEAL PLANNER

WEEK ________________

| Monday |
| Tuesday |
| Wednesday |
| Thursday |
| Friday |
| Saturday |
| Sunday |

To Do List

- ☐ _________________
- ☐ _________________
- ☐ _________________
- ☐ _________________
- ☐ _________________
- ☐ _________________
- ☐ _________________
- ☐ _________________
- ☐ _________________
- ☐ _________________
- ☐ _________________
- ☐ _________________

Notes

____

SEVEN DAY MEAL PLANNER

WEEK _______________

Monday

Tuesday

Wednesday

Thursday

Friday

Saturday

Sunday

To Do List

☐ ___________________
☐ ___________________
☐ ___________________
☐ ___________________
☐ ___________________
☐ ___________________
☐ ___________________
☐ ___________________
☐ ___________________
☐ ___________________
☐ ___________________
☐ ___________________

Notes

____
____
____
____
____
____
____
____
____

SEVEN DAY MEAL PLANNER

WEEK _______________

Monday

Tuesday

Wednesday

Thursday

Friday

Saturday

Sunday

To Do List

- ☐ _______________
- ☐ _______________
- ☐ _______________
- ☐ _______________
- ☐ _______________
- ☐ _______________
- ☐ _______________
- ☐ _______________
- ☐ _______________
- ☐ _______________
- ☐ _______________
- ☐ _______________

Notes

____

SEVEN DAY MEAL PLANNER

WEEK _______________

Monday

Tuesday

Wednesday

Thursday

Friday

Saturday

Sunday

To Do List

- ☐ ___________________
- ☐ ___________________
- ☐ ___________________
- ☐ ___________________
- ☐ ___________________
- ☐ ___________________
- ☐ ___________________
- ☐ ___________________
- ☐ ___________________
- ☐ ___________________
- ☐ ___________________
- ☐ ___________________

Notes

____
____
____
____
____
____
____
____
____

SEVEN DAY MEAL PLANNER

WEEK __________

Monday	To Do List
	☐ ______
Tuesday	☐ ______
	☐ ______
Wednesday	☐ ______
	☐ ______
Thursday	☐ ______
	☐ ______
Friday	☐ ______
	☐ ______
Saturday	☐ ______
	☐ ______
Sunday	☐ ______

Notes

SEVEN DAY MEAL PLANNER

WEEK _______________

Monday

Tuesday

Wednesday

Thursday

Friday

Saturday

Sunday

To Do List

- ☐ _______________
- ☐ _______________
- ☐ _______________
- ☐ _______________
- ☐ _______________
- ☐ _______________
- ☐ _______________
- ☐ _______________
- ☐ _______________
- ☐ _______________
- ☐ _______________
- ☐ _______________

Notes

____

SEVEN DAY MEAL PLANNER

WEEK ______________

Monday

Tuesday

Wednesday

Thursday

Friday

Saturday

Sunday

To Do List

- ☐ ________________
- ☐ ________________
- ☐ ________________
- ☐ ________________
- ☐ ________________
- ☐ ________________
- ☐ ________________
- ☐ ________________
- ☐ ________________
- ☐ ________________
- ☐ ________________
- ☐ ________________

Notes

____
____
____
____
____
____
____
____
____
____

SEVEN DAY MEAL PLANNER

WEEK __________

Monday

Tuesday

Wednesday

Thursday

Friday

Saturday

Sunday

To Do List

- ☐ __________
- ☐ __________
- ☐ __________
- ☐ __________
- ☐ __________
- ☐ __________
- ☐ __________
- ☐ __________
- ☐ __________
- ☐ __________
- ☐ __________
- ☐ __________

Notes

____

SEVEN DAY MEAL PLANNER

WEEK _______________

Monday

Tuesday

Wednesday

Thursday

Friday

Saturday

Sunday

To Do List

- ☐ ___________________
- ☐ ___________________
- ☐ ___________________
- ☐ ___________________
- ☐ ___________________
- ☐ ___________________
- ☐ ___________________
- ☐ ___________________
- ☐ ___________________
- ☐ ___________________
- ☐ ___________________
- ☐ ___________________

Notes

____
____
____
____
____
____
____
____
____

SEVEN DAY MEAL PLANNER

WEEK ___________________

Monday

Tuesday

Wednesday

Thursday

Friday

Saturday

Sunday

To Do List

- ☐ ______________________
- ☐ ______________________
- ☐ ______________________
- ☐ ______________________
- ☐ ______________________
- ☐ ______________________
- ☐ ______________________
- ☐ ______________________
- ☐ ______________________
- ☐ ______________________
- ☐ ______________________
- ☐ ______________________

Notes

____
____
____
____
____
____
____
____
____

SEVEN DAY MEAL PLANNER

WEEK _______________

Monday

Tuesday

Wednesday

Thursday

Friday

Saturday

Sunday

To Do List

- ☐ _______________
- ☐ _______________
- ☐ _______________
- ☐ _______________
- ☐ _______________
- ☐ _______________
- ☐ _______________
- ☐ _______________
- ☐ _______________
- ☐ _______________
- ☐ _______________
- ☐ _______________

Notes

____

____

____

____

____

____

____

____

____

SEVEN DAY MEAL PLANNER

WEEK _____________

Monday

Tuesday

Wednesday

Thursday

Friday

Saturday

Sunday

To Do List

- ☐ _______________
- ☐ _______________
- ☐ _______________
- ☐ _______________
- ☐ _______________
- ☐ _______________
- ☐ _______________
- ☐ _______________
- ☐ _______________
- ☐ _______________
- ☐ _______________
- ☐ _______________

Notes

____

SEVEN DAY MEAL PLANNER

WEEK _____________

Monday

Tuesday

Wednesday

Thursday

Friday

Saturday

Sunday

To Do List

- ☐ _______________
- ☐ _______________
- ☐ _______________
- ☐ _______________
- ☐ _______________
- ☐ _______________
- ☐ _______________
- ☐ _______________
- ☐ _______________
- ☐ _______________
- ☐ _______________
- ☐ _______________
- ☐ _______________

Notes

____

SEVEN DAY MEAL PLANNER

WEEK _____________

Monday	To Do List
Tuesday	☐ _____________
Wednesday	☐ _____________
Thursday	☐ _____________
Friday	☐ _____________
Saturday	Notes
Sunday